MIXER DESSERTS COOKBOOK

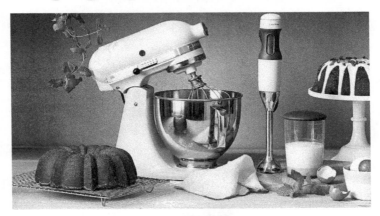

FOR BEGINNERS

Dylan Lambert

Table of Contents

3

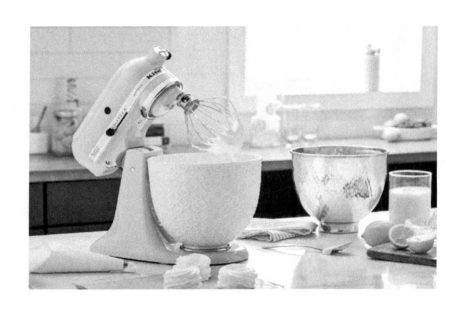

Chocolate Hazelnut Praline Torte With Frangelico Whipped Cream

Serving: Makes 1 torte | Prep: | Cook: | Ready in:

<u>Ingredients</u>

- 1 recipeHazelnut Praline

- 3 ounces fine-quality bittersweet chocolate (not unsweetened), chopped coarse

- 3/4 stick (6 tablespoons) unsalted butter, softened

- 1 teaspoon salt

- 1/2 cup sugar

- 4 large eggs, separated

- 1 teaspoon vanilla extract

- 1 cup well-chilled heavy cream

- 2 tablespoons Frangelico (hazelnut-flavored liqueur)

Direction

1. Preheat an oven to 350°F. Butter the 8 1/2-in., 2-in. deep springform pan/other cake pan with the same dimensions; line wax paper round on bottom. Butter paper. Use flour to dust pan; knock excess flour out.

2. Pulse praline till ground fine in a food processor; keep 1/4 cup ground praline. Put leftover praline into a bowl. Pulse chocolate till finely ground in a food processor; add to bowl with praline.

3. Cream 1/4 cup sugar, salt and butter using an electric mixer till fluffy and light in a bowl. One by one, beat in yolks; beat well after each. Then beat in the vanilla. Mix in praline chocolate mixture; it'll be very thick.

4. Beat whites using cleaned beaters till foamy in another bowl. In a stream, add leftover 1/4 cup sugar and pinch salt, beating till meringue

holds stiff peaks. Fold 1/3 meringue to lighten into yolk mixture; gently yet thoroughly fold in leftover meringue. Put batter in pan; smooth top.

5. Bake torte in center of oven till it starts to pull away from pan's sides for 45-55 minutes. In pan on rack, cool torte; it'll slightly fall and sets as it cooks. Remove from pan. You can make it 1 day ahead, covered, chilled. Before serving, bring to room temperature.

6. Beat cream with an electric mixer in a bowl just until soft peaks hold. Mix in 1/2 reserved praline and Frangelico.

7. Put whipped cream on torte; sprinkle leftover reserved praline. Immediately serve.

Chocolate Layer Cake With Mocha Frosting And Almonds

Serving: Makes 12 servings | Prep: | Cook: | Ready in:

Ingredients

- 1 1/4 cups cake flour

- 3/4 teaspoon baking soda

- 1/4 teaspoon salt

- 1 1/3 cups sugar

- 1/3 cup unsweetened cocoa powder

- 2/3 cup buttermilk

- 1 teaspoon vanilla extract

- 10 tablespoons (1 1/4 sticks) unsalted butter, room temperature

- 1 large egg

- 1 large egg yolk

- 1 tablespoon instant espresso powder or coffee crystals

- 2 teaspoons vanilla extract

- 10 ounces semisweet chocolate, chopped

- 1 cup (2 sticks) unsalted butter, room temperature

- 1 tablespoon light corn syrup

- 2 cups powdered sugar, sifted

- 1 cup sliced almonds, lightly toasted

<u>Direction</u>

1. Cake: In middle of oven, put rack; preheat to 350°F. Line parchment paper on bottom of 9-in. round cake pan that has 2-in. high sides. Butter and flour parchment and sides of pan. Sift salt, baking soda and flour into medium bowl. Whisk cocoa and 2/3 cup sugar to blend in another medium bowl. Add vanilla and 1/3 cup buttermilk; whisk till smooth. Beat butter using electric mixer till fluffy in big bowl. Add

2/3 cup of sugar; beat till blended well. Beat in egg yolk and egg. Add buttermilk-cocoa mixture and beat to blend. In 3 additions and alternately with 1/3 cup of buttermilk in 2 additions, beat in flour mixture; put batter in pan.

2. Bake cake for 40 minutes till inserted tester in middle exits clean; cool cake for 30 minutes in pan on rack. Around pan sides, cut; invert cake on plate. Peel parchment paper off.

3. Frosting: Mix vanilla and espresso powder till espresso melts in small bowl. Mix chocolate till smooth and melted on top of double boiler above simmering water. Take from above water; cool. Beat butter using electric mixer till fluffy in big bowl. Add corn syrup and espresso mixture; blend well, occasionally scraping down bowl's sides. Beat in melted chocolate; in 3 additions, beat in powdered sugar. Freeze till firm to spread, occasionally mixing, for 10 minutes if the frosting is very soft.

4. Put 2/3 cup frosting in pastry bag with medium star tip. Horizontally halve cake. Put bottom layer onto 8-in. cardboard round/8-in. tart pan bottom. On bottom cake layer, spread 1 cup frosting. Put 2nd cake layer over; spread leftover frosting on sides and top of cake. Put 24 almond slices aside. Press leftover almonds on cake's sides. Around cake's top edge, pipe 12 frosting rosettes, spacing evenly. In each rosette, put 2 almond slices. You can make it 1 day ahead, chilled, covered. Stand 2 hours before serving at room temperature.

Nutrition Information

- Calories: 611
- Saturated Fat: 21 g(104%)
- Sodium: 318 mg(13%)
- Fiber: 4 g(14%)
- Total Carbohydrate: 71 g(24%)
- Cholesterol: 98 mg(33%)

Chocolate Mint Mousse

Serving: Makes 4 servings | Prep: 15mins | Cook: 1.75hours | Ready in:

Ingredients

- 1 1/3 cups chilled heavy cream

- 5 oz fine-quality bittersweet chocolate (no more than 60% cacao if marked), finely chopped

- 1/2 teaspoon pure peppermint extract

- 1/2 cup coarsely crushed peppermint hard candies (2 oz)

Direction

1. Over low heat, heat in a 1-quart saucepan the 1/3 cup of cream until hot. Add in chocolate and a pinch of salt then whisk until smooth. Prepare bowl and place mixture. Allow cooling

at room temperature for about 30 minutes while occasionally stirring.

2. In a separate bowl, set an electric mixer at medium speed and whisk the rest of the cream with extract until it holds soft peaks. Pour in cooled chocolate mixture and whisk until mousse holds stiff peaks. Add 1/4 cup of candy; fold. Scoop into 4 stemmed glasses and sprinkle with the rest of 1/4 cup candy. Place in the chiller for about 1 hour until cold.

Nutrition Information

- Calories: 410
- Protein: 9 g(17%)
- Total Fat: 34 g(53%)
- Saturated Fat: 21 g(106%)
- Sodium: 43 mg(2%)
- Fiber: 13 g(52%)
- Total Carbohydrate: 37 g(12%)
- Cholesterol: 109 mg(36%)

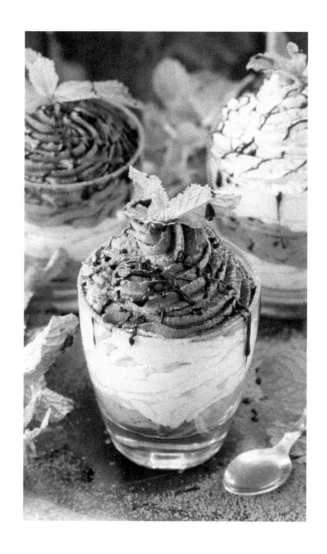

Chocolate Orange Cheesecake With Orange Tangerine Glaze

Serving: Serves 8 | Prep: | Cook: | Ready in:

Ingredients

- about 30 chocolate wafers, ground fine in a blender or food processor (1 3/4 cups)

- 1/2 stick (1/4 cup) unsalted butter, melted

- 1 1/2 pounds cream cheese, softened

- 1 1/4 cups sugar

- 1 cup sour cream at room temperature

- 2 tablespoons freshly grated orange zest (from about 4 navel oranges)

- 1/4 cup plus 2 tablespoons fresh orange juice

- 2 tablespoons Grand Marnier or other orange-flavored liqueur

- 1/2 teaspoon salt

- 1/4 cup all-purpose flour

- 4 large whole eggs

- 1 large egg yolk

- 3/4 cup orange and tangerine marmalade* (about 7 1/2 ounces)

- *available at some specialty food shops.

Direction

1. For Crust: Mix butter and wafer crumbs till well combined in a small bowl; pat crumb mixture 1-in. up the side and on bottom of 9-in. springform pan. Chill crust for 30 minutes.

2. For Filling: Preheat an oven to 300°F.

3. Beat cream cheese till fluffy and light using an electric mixer in a bowl; slowly beat in sugar till well combined. Beat in flour, salt, liqueur, orange juice, zest and sour cream. Beat in yolk

and whole egg, one at a time; beat well after each addition.

4. Wrap side and bottom of springform pan, one at a time, using three 14x12-in. foil pieces, putting every piece in a different position to make sure that the foil is at least 1 1/2-in. up the side all around. In big baking dish, put pan; pour filling into the crust. Put dish in center of oven; slowly add water with a measuring cup to reach 1/4-in. up springform pan's side. Don't let water get in the foil. Cooling in water bath avoids the cheesecake surface from getting cracks.

5. Bake cheesecake till edges are set yet center slightly trembles, for 1 hour 15 minutes; turn off oven. Allow cheesecake to stand for 1 hour; it sets while standing. Carefully take dish from oven. Put cheesecake in pan onto a rack; fully cool. Remove foil; chill cheesecake for 6 hours – overnight, loosely covered.

6. For Glaze: Melt marmalade on medium heat in a small saucepan, mixing; cool to warm.

7. Remove springform pan's sides; evenly spread marmalade over cheesecake. Chill cheesecake for 2 hours; glaze softens if served in room temperature.

Nutrition Information

- Calories: 610

- Total Fat: 44 g(67%)

- Saturated Fat: 24 g(122%)

- Sodium: 508 mg(21%)

- Fiber: 1 g(3%)

- Total Carbohydrate: 46 g(15%)

- Cholesterol: 240 mg(80%)

- Protein: 10 g(20%)

Chocolate Peppermint Bark Cookies

Serving: Makes about 36 | Prep: | Cook: | Ready in:

Ingredients

- Nonstick vegetable oil spray

- 2 cups all purpose flour

- 1/4 teaspoon salt

- 1 cup (2 sticks) unsalted butter, room temperature

- 1 cup sugar

- 1 teaspoon vanilla extract

- 1 large egg yolk

- 6 ounces bittersweet or semisweet chocolate, chopped

- 1/2 cup finely chopped red-and-whitestriped hard peppermint candies or candy canes (about 3 ounces)

- 2 ounces high-quality white chocolate (such as Lindt or Perugina)

Direction

1. Preheat an oven to 350°F; spray nonstick spray on 13x9x2-in. metal baking pan. Line long 9-in. wide parchment paper strip on bottom of pan; leave overhang over both pan's short sides. Whisk salt and flour in medium bowl. Beat butter using electric mixer for 2 minutes till creamy in big bowl; beat in sugar slowly. Beat till fluffy and light for 3 minutes, occasionally stopping to scrape bowl's sides down. Beat in vanilla; beat in egg yolk. Add flour mixture slowly; beat to just blend on low speed.

2. By tablespoonfuls, drop dough in prepped baking pan, evenly spacing; press dough to make even layer on bottom of pan using

moistened fingertips. Use fork to pierce dough all over.

3. Bake cookie base for 30 minutes till edges start to come away from pan's sides, slightly puffed and light golden brown. Put pan on rack; sprinkle bittersweet chocolate immediately. Sprinkle bittersweet chocolate immediately. Stand for 3 minutes till chocolate softens. Spread bittersweet chocolate in thin even layer on top of cookie using small offset spatula; sprinkle chopped peppermint candies immediately.

4. Mix white chocolate till smooth and melted in medium metal bowl above saucepan of simmering water; discard from over water. Drizzle white chocolate using fork all over cookies. Chill for 30 minutes till white chocolate sets.

5. Lift cookie from pan using paper overhang for aid; put onto work surface. Cut cookie to irregular pieces using big knife. You can make it 1 week ahead; keep in airtight containers

between wax paper/parchment paper layers in airtight containers.

6. Variation: Sprinkle chopped peanut brittle/peanut butter cups with melted dark chocolate instead of peppermint candies.

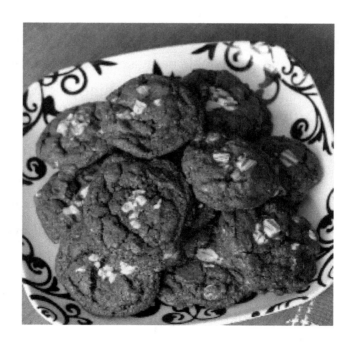

Chocolate Cherry Tart

Serving: Makes 10 to 12 servings | Prep: | Cook: |
Ready in:

Ingredients

- 1/2 cup water

- 1/2 cup sugar

- 1 cup (packed) dried Bing (sweet) cherries

- 1/3 cup kirsch (clear cherry brandy)

- 1 cup (2 sticks) unsalted butter, room temperature

- 1/2 cup sugar

- 1 large egg

- 1 teaspoon vanilla extract

- 2 cups all purpose flour

- 5 tablespoons unsweetened cocoa powder

- 1/2 teaspoon salt

- 3 large eggs

- 1/3 cup dark corn syrup

- 1/4 cup (1/2 stick) unsalted butter, melted

- 1 teaspoon vanilla extract

- 1/2 teaspoon (scant) salt

- 1/2 cup sugar

- 6 ounces bittersweet (not unsweetened) or semisweet chocolate, chopped

- Powdered sugar

- Unsweetened cocoa powder

Direction

1. Fruit: Mix sugar and 1/2 cup water till syrup boils and sugar is dissolved in medium heavy saucepan on medium heat. Add cherries; take off heat. Cool for 30 minutes. Stir in kirsch; cover. Refrigerate for 1 day.

2. Crust: Beat butter using electric mixer till fluffy in big bowl. Add sugar; beat till smooth. Beat in vanilla and egg. Sift salt, cocoa and flour on top; beat to blend. Press dough with moistened fingertips up sides and on bottom of 11-in. diameter tart pan that has removable bottom; cover. Chill for a minimum of 1 hour – maximum of 1 day.

3. Filling: Preheat an oven to 350°F. Drain the cherries; keep cherry syrup. In crust, sprinkle cherries. Mix salt, vanilla, butter, corn syrup and eggs in big bowl. Add 1/4 cup sherry syrup and sugar; beat to blend. Stir in chocolate; put filling in crust.

4. Bake tart for 1 hour till set in center; cool for 30 minutes on rack. You can make it 1 day ahead; cover. Keep in room temperature. From pan, release tart. Dust cocoa and powdered sugar; serve at room temperature/warm.

Nutrition Information

- Calories: 594

- Fiber: 3 g(12%)

- Total Carbohydrate: 74 g(25%)

- Cholesterol: 135 mg(45%)

- Protein: 7 g(13%)

- Total Fat: 31 g(47%)

- Saturated Fat: 18 g(92%)

- Sodium: 285 mg(12%)

Chocolate Chocolate Chip Cookie And Strawberry Gelato Sandwiches

Serving: Makes about 12 sandwiches | Prep: | Cook: |
Ready in:

Ingredients

- 2 1/4 cups all purpose flour

- 1/2 cup natural unsweetened cocoa powder

- 1 teaspoon baking soda

- 1/2 teaspoon salt

- 1 cup (2 sticks) unsalted butter, room temperature

- 1 cup (packed) dark brown sugar

- 1/2 cup sugar

- 2 large eggs

- 1 teaspoon vanilla extract

- 1/2 teaspoon almond extract

- 2 cups semisweet chocolate chips

- Fresh Strawberry Gelato , slightly softened

Direction

1. Preheat an oven to 375°F; line parchment on 2 big rimmed baking sheets. Sift initial 4 ingredients into bowl. Beat butter using electric mixer till fluffy in big bowl. Beat in both sugars; one by one, beat in eggs. Beat in extracts; beat in flour mixture. Fold in the chocolate chips. By heaping tablespoonfuls, drop batter on prepped sheets, with mounds 2-3-in. apart. Flatten mounds to 3/4-in. thick using moist fingertips.

2. Bake cookies for 5 minutes. Reverse the sheets; bake for 5 minutes till soft to touch yet cookies look dry and are puffed. Fully cool. Freeze for 15 minutes on sheets.

3. On 1 cookie's flat side, put 1/3 cup gelato; put 2nd cookie, flat side down, on top. Press

together. Wrap; freeze. Repeat with leftover cookies and gelato. DO AHEAD: keep for maximum of 48 hours, frozen.

Nutrition Information

- Calories: 483

- Total Carbohydrate: 65 g(22%)

- Cholesterol: 72 mg(24%)

- Protein: 6 g(11%)

- Total Fat: 26 g(39%)

- Saturated Fat: 15 g(77%)

- Sodium: 225 mg(9%)

- Fiber: 4 g(15%)

Chocolate Cinnamon Bundt Cake With Mocha Icing

Serving: Makes 12 to 16 servings | Prep: 20mins | Cook: 1hours35mins | Ready in:

Ingredients

- 1 cup boiling water

- 1/2 cup natural unsweetened cocoa powder

- 4 teaspoons instant espresso powder, divided

- 2 cups unbleached all purpose flour

- 2 teaspoons baking powder

- 2 teaspoons ground cinnamon

- 1 teaspoon salt

- 2 1/2 cups (packed) golden brown sugar, divided

- 1 cup vegetable oil

- 1 tablespoon vanilla extract

- 2 large eggs

- 1 1/4 cups mini semisweet chocolate chips, divided

- 1/4 cup (1/2 stick) unsalted butter, room temperature

Direction

1. Preheat an oven to 350°F. Brush oil on 12-15-cup nonstick Bundt pan generously. Whisk 2 tsp. espresso powder, cocoa powder and 1 cup boiling water in 2-cup glass measure. Whisk salt, cinnamon, baking powder and 2 cups flour in medium bowl. Beat 1 tbsp. vanilla, 1 cup vegetable oil and 2 cups brown sugar using an electric mixer to blend in big bowl. Add eggs and beat to blend; beat for 30 seconds till smooth. Beat in 1/2 of flour mixture; beat in cocoa mixture. Add leftover flour mixture and beat to blend. Fold in the 1

cup chocolate chips; pour batter in prepped Bundt pan.

2. Bake cake for 50 minutes till inserted tester near the middle exits clean; cool cake for 10 minutes. Onto rack, invert cake; cool for 15 minutes.

3. Meanwhile, mix 2 tbsp. water, 2 tsp. espresso powder and leftover 1/2 cup brown sugar till sugar melts in small saucepan on medium heat; remove from heat. Add leftover 1/4 cup chocolate chips and butter; mix till chocolate and butter melt. Slightly cool. Drizzle icing on cake using spoon; fully cool cake. Slice; serve.

-

Chocolate Orange Biscotti

Serving: Makes about 3 dozen | Prep: | Cook: | Ready in:

Ingredients

- 2 cups plus 2 tablespoons all purpose flour

- 1 1/2 teaspoons baking powder

- 1/4 teaspoon salt

- 3/4 cup sugar

- 1/2 cup (1 stick) unsalted butter, room temperature

- 2 large eggs

- 2 tablespoons Grand Marnier or other orange liqueur

- 1 tablespoon grated orange peel

- 1 cup pecans, lightly toasted, coarsely chopped

- 6 ounces bittersweet (not unsweetened) chocolate, chopped

Direction

1. Line parchment paper on big baking sheet. Whisk salt, baking powder and flour to blend in medium bowl. Beat butter and sugar using electric mixer to blend in big bowl. One by one, beat in eggs then orange peel and Grand Marnier. Add flour mixture; beat till blended. Mix in chocolate and pecans. Gather dough together; halve. Wrap in plastic; freeze to firm for 20 minutes.

2. In middle of oven, put rack; preheat it to 350°F. Form each dough piece to 2 1/2-in. wide, 14-in. long log using floured hands. Put logs on prepped baking sheet, 2-in. apart; bake for 30 minutes till light golden. Put parchment on rack with logs; cool for 20 minutes. Lower oven temperature down to 300°F.

3. On cutting board, put 1 log; on diagonal, cut log to 1/2-in. thick slices using serrated knife;

stand slices on baking sheet, upright. Repeat with leftover log.

4. Bake biscotti for 30 minutes till pale golden and dry to touch; on rack, fully cool. You can make it 1 week ahead; keep in airtight container.

Nutrition Information

- Calories: 314
- Cholesterol: 44 mg(15%)
- Protein: 5 g(11%)
- Total Fat: 19 g(29%)
- Saturated Fat: 9 g(44%)
- Sodium: 95 mg(4%)
- Fiber: 3 g(13%)
- Total Carbohydrate: 31 g(10%)

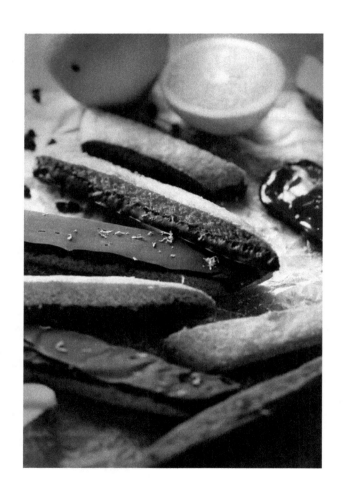

Chocolate Orange Carrot Cake

Serving: Serves 8 to 10 | Prep: | Cook: | Ready in:

Ingredients

- Nonstick vegetable oil spray

- 1 1/2 cups vegetable oil

- 4 large eggs

- 2 1/2 cups all purpose flour

- 2 1/4 cups sugar

- 2/3 cup unsweetened cocoa powder

- 2 teaspoons baking soda

- 1 teaspoon salt

- 2 cups finely shredded peeled carrots (about 10 ounces)

- 1 cup (packed) sweetened flaked coconut

- 1 1/2 teaspoons grated orange peel

- 1 11-ounce can mandarin oranges, drained, cut into 1/2-inch pieces

- 2 1/2 cups semisweet chocolate chips (about 15 ounces)

- 1 cup (2 sticks) unsalted nondairy (pareve) margarine, room temperature

- 1/3 cup powdered sugar

- 1/4 cup frozen orange juice concentrate, thawed

- Additional canned mandarin orange segments, drained, patted very dry

Direction

1. Cake: Preheat an oven to 350°F. Spray nonstick spray on 2 9-in. diameter cake pans that have 2-in. high sides. Beat eggs and 1 1/2 cups oil using electric mixer for 2 minutes till thick and well blended in big bowl. Add salt, baking soda, cocoa powder, sugar and flour;

beat to blend on low speed. Increase speed; beat for 1 minute. It'll be very thick. Mix in orange peel, coconut, carrots then orange pieces. Divide the batter to prepped pans.

2. Bake cakes for 40 minutes till inserted tester in middle exits clean; cool cakes for 10 minutes in pan. Turn onto racks; fully cool.

3. Frosting: Mix chocolate chips till smooth and melted in medium heavy saucepan on very low heat; take off heat. Cool to lukewarm. Put 1/3 cup chocolate in small bowl; keep for decoration. Beat sugar and margarine till fluffy in medium bowl; beat in orange juice concentrate and leftover melted chocolate.

4. On platter, put 1 cake layer; spread 2/3 cup frosting. Put 2nd cake layer over; spread leftover frosting on sides and top of cake. Put extra orange segments around cake's top edge. Rewarm 1/3 cup of reserved chocolate if needed to pourable consistency; drizzle chocolate on orange segments. You can make

it 1 day ahead. Use a cake dome to cover; refrigerate.

Nutrition Information

- Calories: 1397
- Cholesterol: 93 mg(31%)
- Protein: 12 g(24%)
- Total Fat: 92 g(142%)
- Saturated Fat: 21 g(105%)
- Sodium: 826 mg(34%)
- Fiber: 10 g(39%)
- Total Carbohydrate: 146 g(49%)

Chocolate Orange Decadence

Serving: Serves 12 | Prep: | Cook: | Ready in:

Ingredients

- 2 medium oranges

- 1 1/3 cups sugar

- 1/4 cup orange marmalade

- 3/4 cup (1 1/2 sticks) unsalted butter, room temperature

- 1 teaspoon vanilla extract

- 4 large eggs, room temperature

- 2 1/2 cups cake flour

- 1/2 teaspoon baking powder

- 1/4 teaspoon baking soda

- 3/4 cup orange juice

- 2 1/2 cups whipping cream

- 9 tablespoons unsalted butter

- 30 ounces bittersweet (not unsweetened) or semisweet chocolate,chopped

- 7 tablespoons Grand Marnier or orange juice

- 3 tablespoons thawed frozen orange juice concentrate

- 2 tablespoons minced orange peel

- 6 tablespoons orange marmalade

- 6 tablespoons Grand Marnier or orange juice

- 3 1/2 1/2-pint baskets of raspberries (or 5 1/4 cups frozen unsweetened raspberries, thawed, drained

- Mint sprigs

Direction

1. To make cake: Preheat the oven to 350°F. Butter 2 cake pans with 9 in. diameter and 1 1/2-in.-high sides. Line waxed paper on the

bottoms of the pan. Use a vegetable peeler to discard strips of peel from the orange. In a processor, chop the peel coarsely and stop occasionally to scrap down the bowl's sides. Blend in 1/3 cup of sugar to mince the peel. Place in marmalade and puree. In a large bowl, cream vanilla and pureed mixture with cream butter using an electric mixer till fluffy and light. Add in the leftover 1 cup of sugar and beat. Add 1 egg at a time, beat well after each addition. In a small bowl, sift the dry ingredients then mix into the batter, alternating with orange juice.

2. Place the batter into prepped pans. Bake cakes for 38 minutes till a tester comes out clean after being inserted in the middle and the tops turn golden. Let cakes cool for 10 minutes on racks. Loosen cakes by using a sharp knife to run around sides of the pan. Turn out and place the cakes onto racks to cool. Discard the paper.

3. To make chocolate ganache: In a heavy large saucepan, bring butter and cream to a simmer. Lower to low heat. Stir in chopped chocolate till melted. Add in the leftover ingredients and mix. In a large bowl, place the ganache and let freeze for 1 hour 15 minutes while stirring frequently till very thick but spreadable.

4. To make glaze: In a heavy small saucepan, melt marmalade over low heat. Take away from the heat then add in Grand Marnier and mix.

5. Slice each cake into 2 layers of cake. On a plate, place the first cake later then brush with 1/4 of glaze. Spread over with 1 cup of ganache. Place the second layer on top then brush with 1/4 of glaze. Spread over with 3/4 cup of ganache. Place 1 1/2 baskets (about 2 1/2 cups) of berries on top. Spread over the third layer of cake with 1/2 cup of ganache. Invert over the berries with the chocolate side facing down. Brush with 1/4 of glaze then spread over with 1 cup of ganache. Place the

fourth layer of cake on top and brush with the leftover glaze. Spread over the top of the cake with 3/4 cup of ganache. Add 1 cup of ganache into the pastry bag with medium star top fitted. Spread over the cake's sides with the leftover ganache, draw the icing spatula up for vertical lines. Around the bottom and top edges of the cake, pipe decorative ganache border. Let the cake freeze for 20 minutes. Top the cake with the leftover berries to cover completely. You can prepare this 1 day ahead. Use plastic wrap to loosely cover the cake and store in the fridge.

6. Add mint sprigs for garnish. Serve the cake at room temperature.

Nutrition Information

- Calories: 996
- Sodium: 104 mg(4%)
- Fiber: 8 g(33%)
- Total Carbohydrate: 114 g(38%)

- Cholesterol: 171 mg(57%)

- Protein: 10 g(19%)

- Total Fat: 59 g(91%)

- Saturated Fat: 36 g(178%)

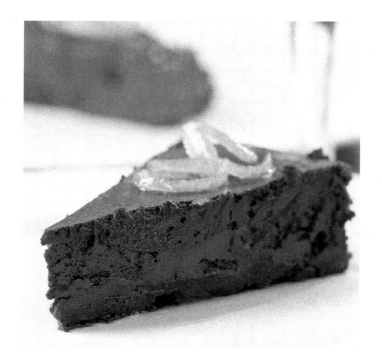

Chocolate Orange Fruitcake With Pecans

Serving: Serves 16 | Prep: | Cook: | Ready in:

Ingredients

- 2 1/2 cups large pecan pieces, toasted

- 1 cup (packed) chopped dried black Mission figs

- 1 cup (packed) chopped pitted prunes

- 1 cup (packed) chopped pitted dates

- 1/2 cup frozen orange juice concentrate, thawed

- 1/4 cup Grand Marnier or other orange liqueur

- 2 tablespoons grated orange peel

- 3 cups all purpose flour

- 3/4 cup (packed) unsweetened cocoa powder

- 2 1/2 teaspoons ground cinnamon

- 1 1/2 teaspoons baking powder

- 1 1/2 teaspoons baking soda

- 1 teaspoon salt

- 1 1-pound box dark brown sugar

- 6 ounces bittersweet (not unsweetened) or semisweet chocolate, coarsely chopped

- 1/2 cup (1 stick) unsalted butter, room temperature

- 4 ounces cream cheese, room temperature

- 4 large eggs, room temperature

- 3/4 cup purchased prune butter

- 1/2 cup plus 2 tablespoons (1 1/4 sticks) unsalted butter

- 1 pound bittersweet (not unsweetened) or semisweet chocolate, chopped

- 6 tablespoons orange juice concentrate, thawed

- Chopped candied fruit peel (optional)

Direction

1. To make cake: Preheat the oven with the rack positioned in the bottom third to 325°F. Generously butter and spread flour on an angel food cake pan with 12 cups. In a large bowl, combine grated orange peel, Grand Marnier, orange juice concentrate, dates, prunes, chopped dried figs and toasted pecans. Allow to stand while stirring occasionally for 30 minutes.

2. In a medium bowl, sift salt, baking soda, baking powder, cinnamon, cocoa and flour. In a processor, combine 6 ounces of chocolate and brown sugar then chop into small pieces.

3. In a large bowl, beat cream cheese and butter by an electric mixer till blended. Beat in chocolate mix till fluffy. Beat in 1 egg at a time. Add in prune butter and beat. Add in 1/4 of dry ingredients and stir. Mix in 3 additions each of the leftover dry ingredients and fruit mixture.

4. Place the batter into the prepped pan. Bake for 1 hour 55 minutes till a tester is attached with a few moist crumbs when being inserted near the middle. Let cool for 5 minutes. Turn then pan over and place onto rack; allow to stand for 5 minutes. Lift off the pan and let the cake cool completely. Use plastic to wrap and keep for 2 days at room temperature.

5. To make glaze: In a heavy medium saucepan, melt butter over low heat. Stir in chocolate till smooth and melted. Add in orange juice concentrate and whisk.

6. Put the cake on rack. Spread thickly over the sides and top of the cakes with some chocolate glaze. Store in the fridge for 15 minutes. Spread over the cake with the leftover glaze to completely cover. If preferred, sprinkle chopped candied fruit peel over. Store the cake for 30 minutes in the fridge till the glaze is set. You can prepare fruitcake for 3 weeks ahead. Use plastic to wrap the cake and store in the fridge.

Nutrition Information

- Calories: 860

- Cholesterol: 111 mg(37%)

- Protein: 10 g(19%)

- Total Fat: 52 g(80%)

- Saturated Fat: 24 g(120%)

- Sodium: 359 mg(15%)

- Fiber: 9 g(35%)

- Total Carbohydrate: 101 g(34%)

Chocolate Peanut Butter Terrine With Sugared Peanuts

Serving: Serves 8 | Prep: | Cook: | Ready in:

Ingredients

- 11 ounces bittersweet chocolate, finely chopped

- 1 ounce (2 tablespoons) unsalted butter

- 6 tablespoons creamy peanut butter

- 4 large egg yolks

- 1/4 cup granulated sugar

- 1 3/4 cups heavy whipping cream

- 4 ounces bittersweet chocolate, finely chopped

- 2 1/2 ounces (5 tablespoons) unsalted butter

- 2 teaspoons light corn syrup

- 1 large egg white

- 6 tablespoons granulated sugar

- 1 1/2 cups (7 1/2 ounces) unsalted peanuts

Direction

1. Terrine: Spray nonstick spray on 8 1/2x4 1/2x2 3/4-in. loaf pan. Line plastic wrap on sprayed pan; leave 1 1/2-in. overhang on all the sides.

2. Mix peanut butter, butter and chocolate in stainless-steel bowl. Put bowl above pan with simmering water; don't let bowl's bottom touch water. Heat till butter and chocolate melt, occasionally mixing. Take from above heat; whisk till smooth.

3. Whip sugar and egg yolks for 1 minute on high speed till thick in a stand mixer's bowl with whip attachment. Take bowl from mixer stand. In 3 even additions, mix in chocolate mixture using wooden spoon; it'll be rather thick.

4. Whisk cream till it begins to thicken in another bowl; fold cream in 4 even additions into

chocolate mixture using a spatula. Spread
batter in prepped pan. Use plastic wrap to
cover, overhanging sides. Refrigerate for a
minimum of 4 hours till firm.

5. Unmold terrine: Fold back plastic wrap; invert
   pan onto wire rack. Pull a plastic wrap's corner
   to release terrine from pan. Lift off pan;
   remove plastic wrap carefully. Line parchment
   paper on a baking sheet; put rack into it. Put
   terrine in the fridge while making glaze.

6. Chocolate glaze: Heat corn syrup, butter and
   chocolate in a stainless-steel bowl above a pan
   with simmering water, without bowl's bottom
   touching water, till butter and chocolate melt,
   occasionally mixing. Take off heat; whisk till
   smooth. Glaze should not be so thin it'll run off
   terrine yet pourable. Sit for 30 minutes in
   room temperature if glaze is too thin.

7. Evenly and slowly put glaze on top of terrine;
   let it evenly stream down sides. Spread glaze to
   fully and smoothly cover terrine using an

offset spatula; refrigerate for 30 minutes till glaze is set.

8. Make sugared peanuts as glaze sets: Preheat an oven to 350°F. Whisk egg white till frothy in a bowl; whisk in sugar. Add peanuts; mix till coated with egg white mixture evenly.

9. Spread peanuts on rimmed baking sheet in 1 layer; put in oven. Toast nuts for 15-20 minutes till golden brown and dry, mixing every 5 minutes.

10. Serve: Put terrine on a serving platter; put sugared peanuts over. Cut terrine using a dry, hot knife.

11. You can make terrine 2 days ahead; keep refrigerated. Sugared peanuts keep in room temperature in airtight container for 1 week.

Nutrition Information

- Calories: 1047

- Cholesterol: 276 mg(92%)

- Protein: 17 g(34%)

- Total Fat: 90 g(138%)

- Saturated Fat: 44 g(220%)

- Sodium: 61 mg(3%)

- Fiber: 6 g(24%)

- Total Carbohydrate: 62 g(21%)

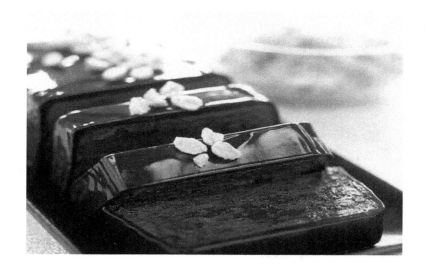

Chocolate Whiskey Truffles Souffles With Caramel Sauce

Serving: Makes 8 servings | Prep: | Cook: | Ready in:

<u>Ingredients</u>

- 3/4 cup whipping cream

- 10 ounces bittersweet (not unsweetened) or semisweet chocolate, chopped

- 1/4 cup whiskey

- 1 1/2 cups whipping cream

- 1 vanilla bean, split lengthwise

- 3/4 cup sugar

- 1/4 cup water

- 4 large eggs, separated

- 1/4 cup plus 2 tablespoons sugar

- 1 1/2 tablespoons cornstarch

- 1 tablespoon unsweetened cocoa powder

- 2/3 cup milk (do not use low-fat or nonfat)

- 4 ounces bittersweet (not unsweetened) or semisweet chocolate, finely chopped

- 1 tablespoon unsalted butter

- 1/2 vanilla bean, split lengthwise

- 1/4 cup whiskey

- Additional sugar (for soufflé dishes)

- Powdered sugar

Direction

1. Making truffles: In a heavy moderate-sized saucepan, add in cream and bring to a boil. Take away from heat. Put in chocolate and whisk until the whole mixture is smooth, also chocolate is melted. Mix whiskey in. Place in the fridge to chill for a minimum of 2 hours, until the mixture is stiff and chilled.

2. Use a tablespoon to drop the truffle mixture on waxed paper. Use foil to line the baking

sheet. Use your palms to roll each chocolate drop (dust your hands with free-sugar cocoa powder in case the truffle sticks to hands). Arrange on baking sheet. Put in the freezer to chill for an hour, until hard then cover it. (You can prepare for 1 week in advance, just keep it frozen)

3. Making sauce: In a small bowl, put in cream. Scratch seeds from vanilla bean then combine bean and seeds into the cream.

4. In a heavy medium saucepan, stir in water and sugar on low heat until sugar has dissolved. Raise the heat and boil the mixture until turns to deep amber color, no stirring. Use damp pastry brush to brush down sides of pan and twirl pan sometimes for 10 minutes. Take away from heat. Put in cream (the mixture will vigorously bubble up). Take the pan back to low heat and stir until caramel is smooth. Keep boiling about 2 minutes until the caramel is thickened and color deepens, while stirring sometimes. Transfer caramel into a small bowl

thorough a strain. Put the sauce in the fridge to chill. (You may prepare sauce 1 week in advance. Cover and keep chilled)

5. Making soufflés: In a medium bowl, blend yolks by whisking then set aside. In a medium stainless steel bowl, stir in cocoa, cornstarch and 1/4 cup sugar until there are not cornstarch lumps anymore. Stir in milk then put in butter and chocolate. Remove seeds from vanilla bean and put bean in.

6. Put chocolate mixture bowl on saucepan of simmering water (do not let the bottom of the bowl touch the water). Whisk for about 2 minutes until the mixture is smooth. Take away from over water. Whisk some hot chocolate mixture gently into yolks. Pour the whisked yolk and chocolate mixture back to chocolate mixture bowl.

7. Put in again over simmering water. Whip for 4 minutes until the mixture thickened and smooth as pudding consistency. Take off from

water. Gently combine in whisky. Get rid of bean. Cool to quite warm.

8. Set the oven to 450°F. Grease eight 2/3- to 3/4-cup custard cups or soufflé dishes with butter. Use sugar to dust all dishes. Place dishes on baking sheet. Put 1 truffle in per dish.

9. In a medium bowl, beat whites by an electric mixer until creating soft peaks. Gently put in 2 tbsp. sugar then beat until firm but not dry.

10. Mix whites into lukewarm soufflé base in 2 additions. Split soufflé mixture among prepared dishes, filling mostly to top. (You can prepare 1 week in advance. Use foil to cover the dish the place in the freezer to chill. Before baking, remove foil to open but do not thaw). Put soufflé on baking sheet in oven. Decrease temperature to 400°F. Bake for 17 minutes if it is unfrozen or 22 minutes if not, until dry-looking on top and puffed.

11. Turn dishes to plates. Drizzle powdered sugar over. Serve while passing separately the chilled caramel sauce.

Nutrition Information

- Calories: 669

- Fiber: 3 g(13%)

- Total Carbohydrate: 70 g(23%)

- Cholesterol: 173 mg(58%)

- Protein: 7 g(15%)

- Total Fat: 40 g(62%)

- Saturated Fat: 24 g(120%)

- Sodium: 74 mg(3%)

Cinnamon Caramel Bread Puddings

Serving: Make 16 servings | Prep: | Cook: | Ready in:

Ingredients

- 20 3 1/2 x 3 1/2-inch slices cinnamon-raisin bread (not ends)

- 12 large eggs

- 2 1/2 cups whole milk

- 2 cups chilled whipping cream, divided

- 1 cup sugar

- 2 tablespoons vanilla extract

- 1 1/2 teaspoons finely grated orange peel

- Pinch of salt

- 2 tablespoons powdered sugar

- Purchased caramel sauce, warmed

Direction

1. Cut bread to 3/4-in. cubes; put into very big bowl. Whisk 1 cup cream, milk, eggs and next 4 ingredients till sugar dissolves in big bowl. Pour egg mixture on bread; toss to coat. Use plastic to cover; to submerge bread in the egg mixture, put a plate on top. Chill for at least 4 hours – overnight.

2. Mix bread mixture; let it stand for 30 minutes at room temperature.

3. Preheat an oven to 375°F. Butter the 16 ramekins or 3/4-cup custard cups; divide to 2 roasting pans and divide bread mixture among cups. Pour hot water in pans until it reaches halfway up sides of cups.

4. Bake puddings for 40 minutes till inserted tester in middle exits clean, edges are golden and puffed; allow puddings to stand for up to 2 hours at room temperature.

5. Beat powdered sugar and leftover 1 cup cream using electric mixer till peaks form in medium

bowl; serve puddings at room
temperature/warm with warm caramel sauce
and whipped cream.

Nutrition Information

- Calories: 310

- Saturated Fat: 8 g(40%)

- Sodium: 225 mg(9%)

- Fiber: 1 g(6%)

- Total Carbohydrate: 34 g(11%)

- Cholesterol: 176 mg(59%)

- Protein: 9 g(18%)

- Total Fat: 15 g(24%)

Citrus Pound Cake

Serving: Makes 8 servings | Prep: 20mins | Cook: 3.5hours | Ready in:

<u>Ingredients</u>

- 2 cups sifted cake flour (not self-rising; sift before measuring)
- 1 teaspoon baking powder
- 1/2 teaspoon salt
- 1 cup granulated sugar
- 1 tablespoon grated orange zest
- 1 teaspoon grated lemon zest
- 2 sticks (1/2 pound) unsalted butter, softened
- 4 large eggs, at room temperature 30 minutes
- 2 teaspoons fresh orange juice
- 1 teaspoon fresh lemon juice
- 1/2 teaspoon pure vanilla extract

- Garnish: confectioners sugar for dusting

<u>Direction</u>

1. Preheat an oven with rack in center to 325°F; butter the 8 1/2x4 1/2-in. loaf pan.

2. Sift salt, baking powder and flour together.

3. Mix zests and sugar using electric mixer on low speed till sugar is colored evenly. Add butter; beat on high speed for 5 minutes till fluffy and pale.

4. One by one, beat in eggs on medium speed, frequently scraping bowl's side down. Beat in vanilla and juices; mix in flour mixture on low speed just till incorporated.

5. In loaf pan, spread batter; rap pan on counter a few times to remove air bubbles. Bake for 1-1 1/4 hours till inserted wooden pick in middle exits clean and golden; cool for 30 minutes in pan on rack. Around pan's edge, run a knife; invert cake onto rack. Fully cool, top side up.

6. Cake improves in flavor if done at least 1 day ahead. You can make it 5 days ahead, kept at room temperature, tightly wrapped.

Nutrition Information

- Calories: 462

- Sodium: 230 mg(10%)

- Fiber: 1 g(3%)

- Total Carbohydrate: 52 g(17%)

- Cholesterol: 154 mg(51%)

- Protein: 6 g(12%)

- Total Fat: 26 g(39%)

- Saturated Fat: 15 g(77%)

Citrus Sponge Cake With Strawberries

Serving: | Prep: | Cook: | Ready in:

Ingredients

- Potato starch (for dusting cake pan)

- 2 teaspoons vegetable oil

- 1/2 cup matzoh cake meal

- 3/4 cup potato starch

- 8 extra-large eggs, separated, at room temperature

- 1 cup sugar

- 1/4 cup orange juice

- Juice of 1 large lemon

- 1 teaspoon freshly grated orange zest

- 1 teaspoon freshly grated lemon zest

- 1 1/2 teaspoons pure vanilla extract

- 1/2 teaspoon almond extract

- 1/4 teaspoon salt

- 3 pints strawberries, stemmed, washed, and thinly sliced

- 1/2 cup orange juice

- 1 tablespoon sugar

Direction

1. Set an oven to 350°F and start preheating. Oil a 9-inch spring form pan lightly, then dust with potato starch.

2. Sift together potato starch and cake meal on a piece of foil, then put aside.

3. Whisk egg yolks in the bowl of an electric mixer at medium speed until thick and golden yellow, for 3 minutes. Slowly put in sugar. Carry on whisking 3 more minutes.

4. Put in gradually lemon zest, orange zest, lemon juice and orange juice using the mixer

at low speed. Put in almond extract and vanilla. Put the matzo meal mixture gradually into the batter. Gently combine until mixed thoroughly.

5. Using the whisk attachment of the electric mixer, whisk egg whites in a clean bowl until foamy. Put in salt and whisk until the whites form glossy peaks. Use a spatula to fold the egg whites into the cake batter gently. Add the batter into the spring form pan and bake until a cake tester comes out clean, or for 50 minutes. In the pan, allow the cake to cool, then loosen the sides. Allow to cool entirely.

6. Slice the cake into twelve wedges or halve the cake horizontally carefully using a serrated knife and slice into six wedges to have 12 wedges in total.

7. Half an hour before serving the cake, toss orange juice and sugar together with strawberries. Scoop strawberries on top of each cake wedge, then serve.

8. Tip: Serve the cake with ice cream or whipped cream to gild the lily.

Nutrition Information

- Calories: 249
- Saturated Fat: 1 g(7%)
- Sodium: 124 mg(5%)
- Fiber: 3 g(10%)
- Total Carbohydrate: 44 g(15%)
- Cholesterol: 167 mg(56%)
- Protein: 7 g(14%)
- Total Fat: 6 g(9%)

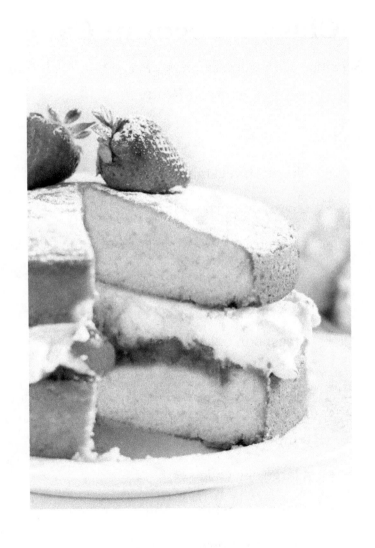

Classic Coconut Cake

Serving: Makes 10 servings | Prep: 30mins | Cook: 4hours | Ready in:

Ingredients

- Nonstick vegetable oil spray

- 2 cups all purpose flour

- 1 1/3 cups (loosely packed) sweetened flaked coconut

- 1 cup buttermilk

- 1 teaspoon baking soda

- 2 cups sugar

- 1 cup (2 sticks) unsalted butter, room temperature

- 5 large egg yolks

- 4 large egg whites, room temperature

- 3 1/3 cups powdered sugar

- 1 8-ounce package philadelphia-brand cream cheese, room temperature

- 1/2 cup (1 stick) unsalted butter, room temperature

- 2 teaspoons vanilla extract

- 1 cup (about) sweetened flaked coconut

Direction

1. Cake: Preheat an oven to 350°F. Use nonstick spray to coat 2 9-in. diameter cake pans that have 1 1/2-in. high sides; line parchment paper rounds on bottom of pans.

2. In medium bowl, mix coconut and flour. In small bowl, whisk baking soda and buttermilk. Beat butter and sugar using electric mixer for 2 minutes till fluffy and light in big bowl. Add egg yolks; beat to blend. In 3 additions, add flour mixture alternately with the buttermilk using 2 additions; beat to just blend after every addition. Beat 1/4 tsp. salt and egg whites using clean dry beaters till peaks form in

another big bowl. Put 1/3 egg white mixture in batter; fold into batter to just blend. In 2 additions, fold in leftover egg white mixture; divide batter to pans.

3. Bake cakes for 35 minutes till inserted tester in middle exits clean; cool cakes for 10 minutes in pans on racks. Around cake pan's sides, run small sharp knife; invert cake on racks. Peel off parchment carefully; fully cool cakes.

4. Frosting: Beat vanilla, butter, cream cheese and sugar using electric mixer till blended in a big bowl. Put 1 cake layer on plate, flat side up; spread 1 cup frosting. Put 2nd layer on frosting, flat side up, spread frosting atop; spread leftover frosting on sides and top of cake. Sprinkle come coconut on cake's top; pat extra coconut on cake's sides. You can make it 1 day ahead. Use cake dome to cover; refrigerate. 1 hour before serving, stand in room temperature.

Nutrition Information

- Calories: 888

- Fiber: 3 g(11%)

- Total Carbohydrate: 112 g(37%)

- Cholesterol: 191 mg(64%)

- Protein: 8 g(17%)

- Total Fat: 47 g(72%)

- Saturated Fat: 28 g(141%)

- Sodium: 343 mg(14%)

Cocoa Nib, Chocolate, And Citrus Dacquoise

Serving: Makes 12 servings | Prep: | Cook: | Ready in:

<u>Ingredients</u>

- Nonstick vegetable oil spray

- 1 cup powdered sugar

- 1 tablespoon cornstarch

- 3/4 cup cocoa nibs* (about 2 1/2 to 3 ounces), finely ground in spice mill or small coffee grinder

- 1/2 teaspoon coarse kosher salt

- 3/4 cup egg whites (about 6 large)

- 1/4 teaspoon cream of tartar

- 1/4 cup sugar

- Nonstick vegetable oil spray

- 1/2 cup sugar, divided

- 1/4 cup all purpose flour

- 1/4 cup unsweetened cocoa powder

- 1/4 teaspoon baking powder

- 1/8 teaspoon baking soda

- 1/8 teaspoon coarse kosher salt

- 1/3 cup canola oil or other vegetable oil

- 2 large eggs, separated

- 2 tablespoons water

- 1 1/4 cups chilled heavy whipping cream

- 1 8-ounce container mascarpone cheese**

- 1/4 cup powdered sugar

- 2 teaspoons vanilla extract

- 6 ounces bittersweet chocolate, chopped

- 3/4 cup heavy whipping cream

- 3 tablespoons water

- 3 tablespoons unsweetened cocoa powder

- 2 tablespoons light corn syrup

- 3 tablespoons unsalted butter, room temperature

- Blood Orange Marmalade

- Blood orange segments (for garnish)

Direction

1. Meringues: Preheat an oven to 300°F. Use parchment paper to line bottoms of 2 9-in. diameter cake pans that have 1 1/2-in. high sides; spray nonstick spray on parchment. In a medium bowl, sift cornstarch and powdered sugar; whisk in 1/2 tsp. coarse salt and ground cocoa bins. Beat cream of tartar and egg whites till foamy and thick in a big bowl. Putting in 1 tbsp. sugar at a time, whip till stiff yet not dry then fold in the cocoa nib mixture. Divide the meringue, evenly spreading, to prepped pans.

2. Bake meringues for 1 hour then turn heat off. Leave meringues in oven, keeping the oven door closed, to dry overnight (they will slightly deflate).

3. Chocolate chiffon cake: Preheat the oven to 325°F. Use parchment paper to line bottom of 9-in. diameter cake pan that has 2-in. high sides; spray nonstick spray on parchment. Mix 1/4 cup sugar with following 5 ingredients in a medium bowl. Whisk to incorporate.

4. Whisk 2 tbsp. water, egg yolks and 1/3 cup oil to blend in big bowl; mix in the dry ingredients. Beat the egg whites till soft peaks form in another medium bowl. Add leftover 1/4 cup sugar slowly, beating till stiff yet not dry. Fold the whites into the yolk mixture; put batter in prepped pan.

5. Bake cake for 25 minutes till an inserted tester in middle exits clean; cool for 15 minutes in pan. Turn out cake onto rack; peel parchment off. Fully cool. You can make it 1 day ahead. Encase using foil; keep at room temperature.

6. Mascarpone whipped cream: Beat all ingredients in a big bowl just till it holds soft peaks (avoid overbeating, otherwise it'll curdle). Cover; chill for 1-2 hours.

7. Glaze: In a big microwave-safe bowl, put chocolate. In medium heavy saucepan, mix light corn syrup, unsweetened cocoa powder, 3 tbsp. water and heavy whipping cream; whisk on medium heat till just starting to boil and blended. Put mixture on chopped chocolate; stand for 1 minute. Mix till smooth then whisk in butter. Stand glaze for 15-20 minutes till thick enough to spread.

8. Put 1 meringue, flat side down, on platter; spread 1/2 cup of glaze on top. Refrigerate for 30 minutes till chocolate sets firmly. Spread half (1 1/2 cups) mascarpone cream on chilled chocolate; refrigerate for 10 minutes. Put cake layer onto work surface; spread 1/2 cup marmalade over then the leftover mascarpone cream. Put cake layer carefully on top of meringue on platter. Put another meringue with flat side up over assembled cake; spread 1/3 glaze on sides and top of cake in an even, thin layer. Refrigerate for 30 minutes till coating sets.

9. Heat leftover glaze for 5-10 seconds in microwave till just pourable yet not hot. Put glaze on cake carefully, spreading to evenly coat; chill cake for at least 1 hour till glaze sets. You can make cake 3 days ahead. Use a cake dome to cover; keep in refrigerator.

10. Slice cold cake to wedges then serve it with blood orange segments.

Nutrition Information

- Calories: 537
- Total Carbohydrate: 43 g(14%)
- Cholesterol: 114 mg(38%)
- Protein: 6 g(12%)
- Total Fat: 40 g(62%)
- Saturated Fat: 18 g(92%)
- Sodium: 246 mg(10%)
- Fiber: 2 g(8%)

Coconut Cream Pie

Serving: 8 | Prep: 25mins | Cook: 30mins | Ready in:

Ingredients

- 1 cup white sugar
- 1/2 cup all-purpose flour
- 1/4 teaspoon salt
- 3 cups milk
- 4 egg yolks
- 3 tablespoons butter
- 1 1/2 teaspoons vanilla extract
- 1 cup flaked coconut
- 1 (9 inch) pie shell, baked

Direction

1. In a medium saucepan, mix together salt, flour and sugar over medium heat; slowly mix in

milk. Cook and stir over medium heat till bubbly and thick. Decrease heat to low and cook for an additional 2 minutes. Remove pan from the heat.

2. Put a strainer on top a clean mixing bowl; put aside.

3. Slightly beat egg yolks. Pour slowly a cup of hot custard mixture into yolks, whisking constantly. Put the egg mixture back into the saucepan; then bring the entire mixture to a gentle boil. Cook and stir for 2 minutes before removing from heat. Pour the custard through the strainer immediately.

4. Mix coconut, vanilla and butter into the hot mixture. Add hot filling into baked pie crust. Allow to cool and chill in the fridge for about 4 hours, until set.

Nutrition Information

- Calories: 399 calories;
- Total Fat: 18.8

- Sodium: 293

- Total Carbohydrate: 51.1

- Cholesterol: 121

- Protein: 6.9

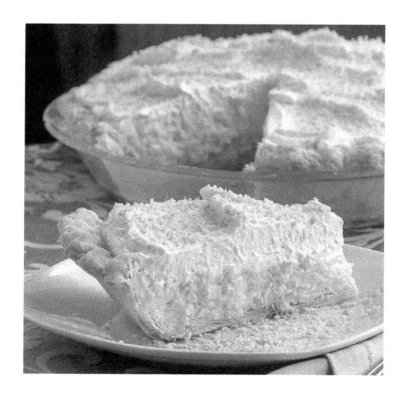

Coconut Cupcakes With White Chocolate Frosting

Serving: Makes 12 cupcakes | Prep: | Cook: | Ready in:

<u>Ingredients</u>

- 1/2 cup coconut cream (not cream of coconut) or milk

- 3 large egg whites

- 1/2 teaspoon pure vanilla extract

- 1 1/2 cups cake flour

- 2 teaspoons baking powder

- 6 tablespoons (3 ounces) unsalted butter, softened

- 1/2 teaspoon salt

- 3/4 cup granulated sugar

- 1/2 cup desiccated or unsweetened coconut, finely ground in a food processor

- 1/2 cup sweetened dried coconut

- 6 ounces white chocolate, finely chopped

- 1 3/4 cups powdered sugar

- 1/4 cup milk

- 4 ounces (8 tablespoons) butter

- 1/2 teaspoon pure vanilla extract

- 1/4 teaspoon salt

Direction

1. Cake: Preheat an oven to 350°F. Put oven rack into center position. Use nonstick spray to coat surface of 12-cup cupcake pan lightly; line paper liner/foil to line each cup.

2. Whisk vanilla extract, egg whites and coconut cream together to combine in a small bowl. Sift baking powder and flour together over parchment paper or in another bowl.

3. Whisk salt and butter till smooth and creamy in an electric mixer with a whisk; in a steady stream, add sugar while beating. Beat for 2-3 minutes at medium speed till fluffy and light, stopping to scrape bowl's sides down as needed.

4. Add 1/3 coconut cream mixture and 1/3 dry ingredients; beat just till combined on low speed. Add leftover coconut cream mixture and dry ingredients in 2 alternation additions, beating between every addition to incorporate fully. Add sweetened dried coconut, final batch of dry ingredients and ground, dried coconut. Scrape bowl down; use a sturdy rubber spatula to mix one more time.

5. Fill each cupcake cup to 2/3 full; knock pan 1-2 times on the countertop to even batter's surface and remove air bubbles. Put pan in oven; rotate pan 180° after 10-12 minutes. Bake till wooden skewer/cake tester exits with crumbs clinging on it and cake springs back

when pressed lightly in the middle. Total baking time is around 20-22 minutes.

6. Cool pan for 5 minutes on a cooling rack. Transfer cookies from pan onto rack; fully cool.

7. Frosting: In a bowl, melt white chocolate above a saucepan of barely simmering water; be sure the bowl's bottom rests a few inches above water's surface. Mix chocolate till smooth; cool on countertop to room temperature.

8. Sift powdered sugar into medium-sized bowl; mix in milk using a whisk till it is smooth and all sugar dissolves. Add salt, vanilla extract and butter; beat till shiny and smooth. Mix in cooled white chocolate with a rubber spatula.

9. Put frosting into the fridge for 30 minutes till cool enough to frost cupcakes; you can keep it for 1 day in room temperature/in the fridge. Before spreading, softened refrigerated frosting in room temperature.

Nutrition Information

- Calories: 458

- Fiber: 1 g(5%)

- Total Carbohydrate: 56 g(19%)

- Cholesterol: 39 mg(13%)

- Protein: 4 g(8%)

- Total Fat: 25 g(39%)

- Saturated Fat: 18 g(88%)

- Sodium: 249 mg(10%)

Coconut Flans

Serving: Makes 8 | Prep: | Cook: | Ready in:

Ingredients

- 2 tablespoons vegetable oil

- 1 tablespoon plus 1/4 cup water

- 1 3/4 cups sugar

- 3/4 cup sweetened flaked coconut

- 1 13.5-ounce can unsweetened coconut milk

- 1 cup whole milk

- 1 vanilla bean, split lengthwise in half

- 8 large egg yolks

- 3 tablespoons triple sec

Direction

1. Whisk 1 tbsp. water and oil to blend in small bowl; brush oil mixture inside 8

ramekins/3/4-cup custard cups. Mix leftover 1/4 cup water and 1 cup sugar in medium heavy saucepan on medium low heat till sugar is dissolved; boil without mixing for 9 minutes till syrup becomes deep amber color, brushing pan sides down with wet pastry brush, swirling sometimes. Divide caramel to prepped custard cups immediately; tilt each custard cup using oven mitts to coat bottom in caramel. Put cups in big roasting pan.

2. Preheat an oven to 350°F. On baking sheet, spread coconut; toast in oven for 10 minutes till light golden, occasionally mixing. Maintain the oven temperature.

3. Mix milk and coconut milk in another medium saucepan. From vanilla bean, scrape in seeds; add bean. Boil; take off heat. Cover; steep for 10 minutes. Discard vanilla bean. Beat 3/4 cup sugar and egg yolks using electric mixer for 4 minutes till pale and thick in big bowl; whisk hot milk mixture slowly into egg mixture then

whisk in triple sec. Mix in 1/2 cup of toasted coconut.

4. Divide custard to caramel-lined custard cups. To reach halfway up custard cup's sides, put hot water in roasting pan; bake for 50 minutes till custards only slightly move when cups are gently shaken and are nearly set; take custards from water. Slightly cool; chill overnight, uncovered.

5. Around custards, run small sharp knife to loosen. Put plate on custard cup to unmold each custard. Grasp plate and custard cup filmy; invert, gently shaking, letting custard settle onto plate. Sprinkle leftover 1/4 cup toasted coconut on custards; serve.

Nutrition Information

- Calories: 426

- Cholesterol: 188 mg(63%)

- Protein: 5 g(10%)

- Total Fat: 21 g(33%)

- Saturated Fat: 14 g(68%)

- Sodium: 52 mg(2%)

- Fiber: 1 g(3%)

- Total Carbohydrate: 53 g(18%)

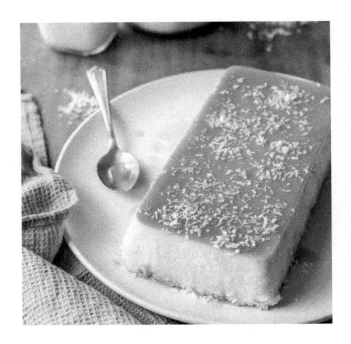

Cornbread Muffins With Maple Butter

Serving: Makes 12 muffins | Prep: | Cook: | Ready in:

Ingredients

- 3/4 cup (1 1/2 sticks) unsalted butter, room temperature
- 3 1/2 tablespoons pure maple syrup (preferably grade B)
- 1 cup yellow cornmeal
- 1 cup unbleached all purpose flour
- 1/4 cup sugar
- 1 tablespoon baking powder
- 1/4 teaspoon salt
- 1 cup buttermilk
- 1 large egg

- 5 tablespoons unsalted butter, melted, cooled slightly

Direction

1. To make maple butter: Use an electric mixer to beat the butter in a medium-sized bowl until it becomes creamy. Slowly beat in the maple syrup until smooth and blended well. You can make this a week ahead, keeping it covered and refrigerated.

2. To make muffins: Heat up an oven to 375 degrees Fahrenheit. Butter 12 regular muffin cups (1/3 cup). In a medium bowl, sieve salt, baking powder, sugar, flour, and cornmeal. In another medium-sized bowl, whisk together egg and buttermilk, then whisk in the melted butter. Add buttermilk mixture into the dry ingredients, stirring until just combined. Be sure not to over-mix. Equally divide the batter into the muffin cups. Bake until a tester is clean once inserted into the center, 15 minutes. The muffins will turn out pale. Cool

the muffins on a rack for 10 minutes, then serve with the maple butter.

Nutrition Information

- Calories: 276
- Cholesterol: 60 mg(20%)
- Protein: 3 g(7%)
- Total Fat: 17 g(26%)
- Saturated Fat: 11 g(53%)
- Sodium: 184 mg(8%)
- Fiber: 1 g(3%)
- Total Carbohydrate: 28 g(9%)

Cornmeal Blini With Tomato Corn Salsa

Serving: Makes 64 | Prep: | Cook: | Ready in:

Ingredients

- 1 cup plus 2 tablespoons low-fat milk

- 2 tablespoons water

- 1/4 cup sugar

- 1 teaspoon dry yeast

- 3/4 cup unbleached all purpose flour

- 2/3 cup yellow cornmeal

- 1 teaspoon salt

- 1/2 cup buttermilk

- 2 large eggs, separated

- 5 teaspoons (about) vegetable oil

- 2 cups frozen corn, thawed, drained

- 1 1/2 pounds tomatoes, seeded, chopped

- 1/2 small red onion, finely chopped

- 6 tablespoons chopped fresh cilantro

- 2 jalapeño chilies, seeded, minced

- 1 tablespoon balsamic vinegar

- 1/2 cup nonfat plain yogurt

Direction

1. Preparing the Blini: In a small saucepan, heat water and milk to room temperature (105 degrees F. to 115 degrees F.). Transfer into a large bowl. Stir in yeast and sugar. Leave to sit for ten minutes.

2. In a medium bowl, mix salt, flour, and cornmeal to blend. Mix into the yeast mixture. Stir in egg yolks and buttermilk. Cover with plastic and allow to sit in a warm spot for about 2 hours until very spongy.

3. In another medium bowl, beat the egg whites using an electric mixer until stiff but not dry.

Carefully roll into the cornmeal mixture in two additions.

4. Preheat an oven to 250 degrees F. Use one teaspoon of oil to rub a large nonstick skillet. Heat on medium-high heat. Work in batches while rubbing with more oil as needed. Transfer the batter by tablespoonfuls into the skillet and spread gently to form 2-inch rounds. Let to cook for about 2 minutes until bubbles start to break on surface and bottoms turn golden. Use a spatula to flip the blini over and let to cook for about 1 minute until golden. Spread onto large baking sheets in a single layer. Place in oven to keep warm.

5. For the Salsa: In a medium bowl, stir all the ingredients apart from yogurt and blend. Add pepper and salt to taste. (You can prepare salsa and blini 8 hours ahead. Then cool the blini. Cover salsa and blini separately and refrigerate. Rewarm the blini while uncovered for about 10 minutes in oven at 350 degrees F prior to serving.)

6. Pour a little amount of yogurt on top of blini. Distribute the salsa on top of blini. Spread onto platters then serve warm.

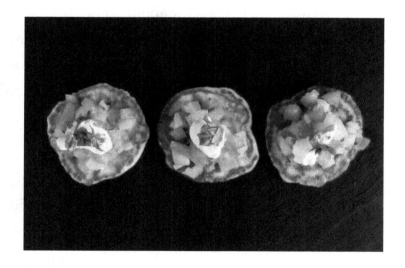

Cornmeal Cake With Sweet Rosemary Syrup And Blackberries

Serving: | Prep: | Cook: | Ready in:

<u>Ingredients</u>

- 1 stick (1/2 cup) unsalted butter, softened

- 1 cup sugar

- 1 cup yellow cornmeal

- 3/4 cup all-purpose flour

- 1 teaspoon baking powder

- 3/4 teaspoon salt

- 2 large eggs

- 1 large egg yolk

- 2/3 cup milk

- Sweet Rosemary Syrup

- lightly sweetened whipped cream
- 2 half-pints blackberries

Direction

1. Cake: Preheat an oven to 350°F. Butter then flour 8x2-in. round cake pan.

2. Beat sugar and butter using electric mixer till fluffy and light in a big bowl. Add leftover cake ingredients; beat till combined on low speed. Beat batter at high speed for 3 minutes till pale yellow.

3. Put batter in prepped pan; bake in center of oven till tester exits with few crumbs adhering for 40 minutes.

4. As cake bakes, make rosemary syrup.

5. Cool cake for 10 minutes in pan on rack. Invert cake onto hand; put on rack, right side up. Brush 1/3 cup syrup slowly on cake while warm, letting syrup soak in then add more. Chill leftover syrup, covered, in a small pitcher. You can make syrup-soaked cake 1 day

ahead; keep in room temperature, wrapped in plastic wrap.

6. Cut cake to wedges; serve with leftover rosemary syrup, blackberries and whipped cream.

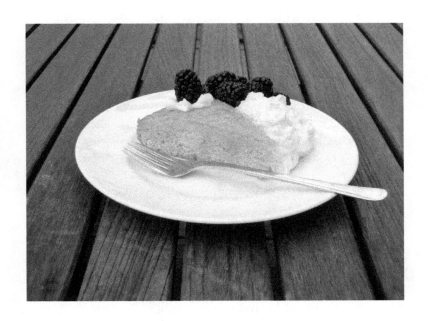

Cornmeal Cookies

Serving: Makes 8 servings | Prep: 20mins | Cook: 2.25hours | Ready in:

Ingredients

- 1 cup yellow cornmeal (not stone-ground)
- 3/4 cup all-purpose flour
- 1/2 teaspoon salt
- 7 tablespoons unsalted butter, softened
- 1/3 cup sugar
- 3/4 teaspoon pure vanilla extract
- 1 large egg plus 1 large egg yolk

Direction

1. Preheat an oven with rack in center to 350°F.
2. Whisk salt, flour and cornmeal. Beat vanilla, sugar and butter using electric mixer on medium speed for 5 minutes till fluffy and

pale, occasionally scraping down bowl's side; beat in yolk and egg till combined well. Lower speed to low. In a slow stream, add cornmeal mixture, mixing just till combined. Shape dough to 5-in. square; chill for 30 minutes till firm while wrapped in a plastic wrap.

3. Roll dough out to 7-in. (1/2-in. thick) square using the lightly floured rolling pin on lightly floured surface; use fork tines to score dough in 1 direction. Cut to 8 even strips, following scored marks; halve strips to make rectangles.

4. Bake for 15-18 minutes on ungreased baking sheet till cookie's bottoms are pale golden. Put on rack; fully cool for 1 hour.

5. You can make cookies 1 day ahead; keep at room temperature in airtight container.

Nutrition Information

- Calories: 254

- Fiber: 1 g(4%)

- Total Carbohydrate: 33 g(11%)

- Cholesterol: 73 mg(24%)

- Protein: 4 g(8%)

- Total Fat: 12 g(18%)

- Saturated Fat: 7 g(34%)

- Sodium: 142 mg(6%)

Chocolate Hazelnut Praline Torte With Frangelico Whipped Cream

Serving: Makes 1 torte | Prep: | Cook: | Ready in:

Ingredients

- 1 recipeHazelnut Praline

- 3 ounces fine-quality bittersweet chocolate (not unsweetened), chopped coarse

- 3/4 stick (6 tablespoons) unsalted butter, softened

- 1 teaspoon salt

- 1/2 cup sugar

- 4 large eggs, separated

- 1 teaspoon vanilla extract

- 1 cup well-chilled heavy cream

- 2 tablespoons Frangelico (hazelnut-flavored liqueur)

Direction

1. Preheat an oven to 350°F. Butter the 8 1/2-in., 2-in. deep springform pan/other cake pan with the same dimensions; line wax paper round on bottom. Butter paper. Use flour to dust pan; knock excess flour out.
2. Pulse praline till ground fine in a food processor; keep 1/4 cup ground praline. Put leftover praline into a bowl. Pulse chocolate till finely ground in a food processor; add to bowl with praline.
3. Cream 1/4 cup sugar, salt and butter using an electric mixer till fluffy and light in a bowl. One by one, beat in yolks; beat well after each. Then beat in the vanilla. Mix in praline chocolate mixture; it'll be very thick.
4. Beat whites using cleaned beaters till foamy in another bowl. In a stream, add leftover 1/4 cup sugar and pinch salt, beating till meringue

holds stiff peaks. Fold 1/3 meringue to lighten into yolk mixture; gently yet thoroughly fold in leftover meringue. Put batter in pan; smooth top.

5. Bake torte in center of oven till it starts to pull away from pan's sides for 45-55 minutes. In pan on rack, cool torte; it'll slightly fall and sets as it cooks. Remove from pan. You can make it 1 day ahead, covered, chilled. Before serving, bring to room temperature.

6. Beat cream with an electric mixer in a bowl just until soft peaks hold. Mix in 1/2 reserved praline and Frangelico.

7. Put whipped cream on torte; sprinkle leftover reserved praline. Immediately serve.

Chocolate Puddings With Orange Whipped Cream

Serving: Makes 6 servings | Prep: 25mins | Cook: 3hours25mins | Ready in:

Ingredients

- 1/2 cup plus 3 tablespoons sugar, divided

- 2 tablespoons cornstarch

- 2 1/2 cups whole milk, divided

- 2 large egg yolks

- 1 1/2 cups bittersweet chocolate chips (do not exceed 61% cacao) or semisweet chocolate chips

- 2 tablespoons (1/4 stick) unsalted butter

- 1/4 teaspoon vanilla extract

- 3/4 cup chilled whipping cream

- 1 tablespoon Grand Marnier or other orange liqueur

- 1/4 teaspoon finely grated orange peel

- Test-kitchen tip: If you don't have orange liqueur on hand, skip the orange peel and use another liqueur. Kahlúa or amaretto would work well in this recipe.

<u>Direction</u>

1. In a medium saucepan, whip cornstarch, quarter teaspoon of salt and half cup plus two tablespoons of sugar to incorporate. Put in egg yolks and half cup of milk; mix till smooth. Mix in the leftover 2 cups of milk. Boil mixture on moderately-high heat, whisk continuously. Boil for a minute, whisk continuously. Take pan off heat; put in butter and chocolate chips. Mix pudding till smooth and melted. Mix in vanilla.

2. Evenly distribute pudding between six wineglasses or dessert cups. Put plastic wrap

right on the top of each to cover pudding fully. Refrigerate for no less than 3 hours, till cold. DO AHEAD: may be done up to one day in advance. Keep in refrigerator.

3. In a medium bowl, whip leftover 1 tablespoon of sugar, orange peel, Grand Marnier and whipping cream with electric mixer to form peaks. DO AHEAD: may be done 2 hours in advance. Refrigerate with cover.

4. Remove puddings cover. Scoop whipped cream dollop on top of each to serve.

Nutrition Information

- Calories: 311
- Protein: 5 g(10%)
- Total Fat: 18 g(28%)
- Saturated Fat: 11 g(53%)
- Sodium: 58 mg(2%)
- Fiber: 0 g(0%)
- Total Carbohydrate: 32 g(11%)

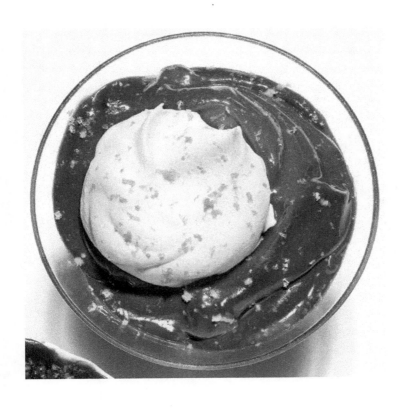

<u>THANK YOU</u>

Thank you for choosing *Mixer Desserts Cookbook for Beginners* for improving your skills! I hope you enjoyed the recipes while making them and tasting them! If you're interested in learning new recipes and new meals to cook, go and check out the other books of the serie.